The Journey of a Beautiful Princess

Ms. Myer

THE JOURNEY OF A BEAUTIFUL PRINCESS

iUniverse books may be ordered through booksellers or by contacting:

iUniverse
1663 Liberty Drive
Bloomington, IN 47403
www.iuniverse.com
1-800-Authors (1-800-288-4677)

Because of the dynamic nature of the Internet, any web addresses or links contained in this book may have changed since publication and may no longer be valid. The views expressed in this work are solely those of the author and do not necessarily reflect the views of the publisher, and the publisher hereby disclaims any responsibility for them.

Any people depicted in stock imagery provided by Getty Images are models, and such images are being used for illustrative purposes only. Certain stock imagery © Getty Images.

ISBN: 978-1-5320-5613-0 (sc)
ISBN: 978-1-5320-5614-7 (e)

Library of Congress Control Number: 2018912388

Print information available on the last page.

iUniverse rev. date: 10/15/2018

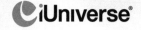

Once upon a time SHINE and baby by the name of FALSE. FALSE is a very smart little girl with hopes and dreams just like any other young girls her age. She will love to do things like modeling or teaching to teach other kids the things she had to go through so early in life....

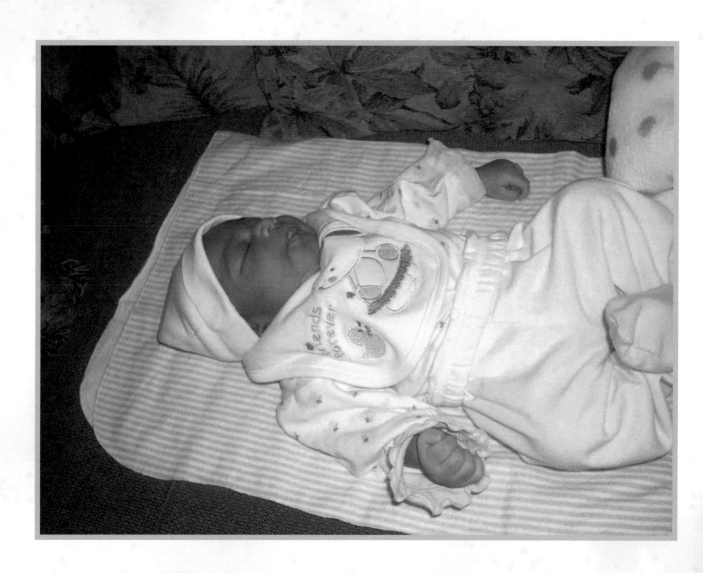

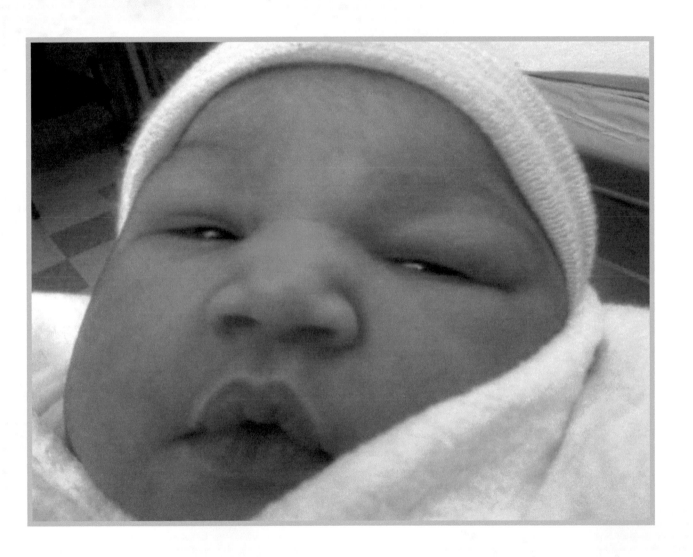

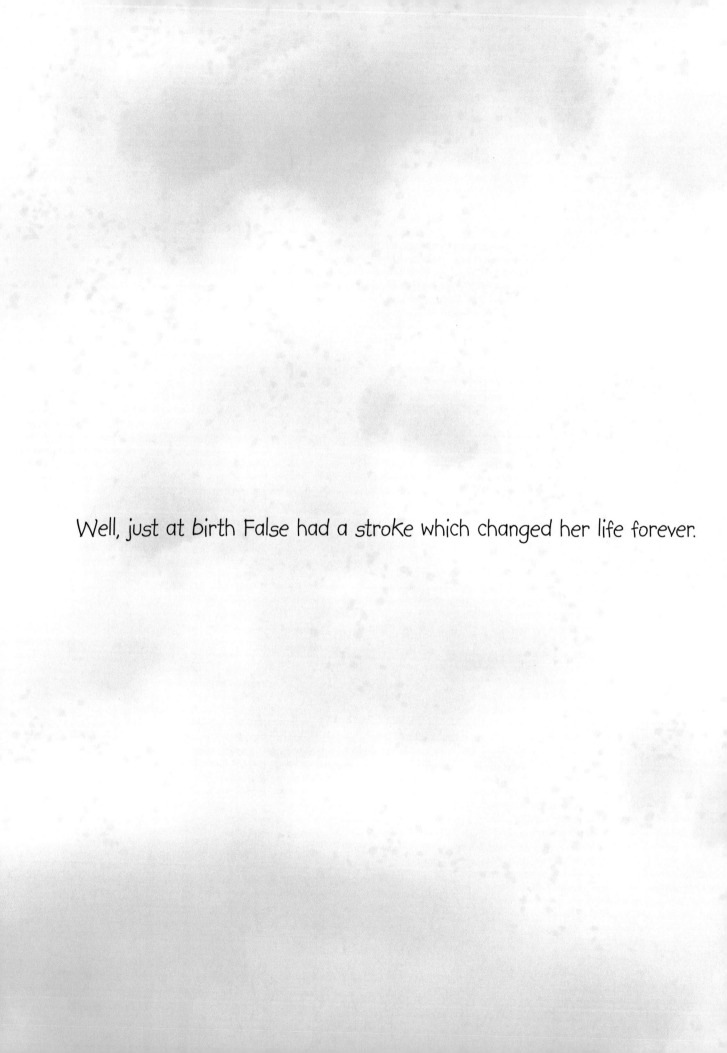

Well, just at birth False had a stroke which changed her life forever.

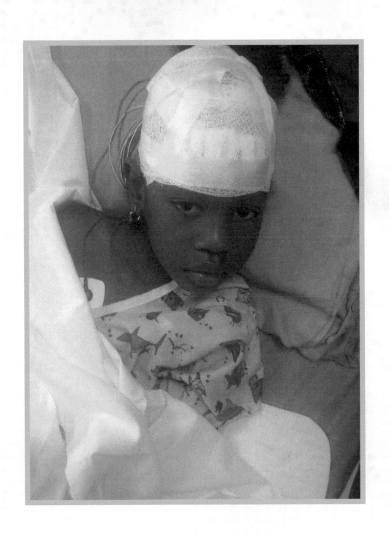
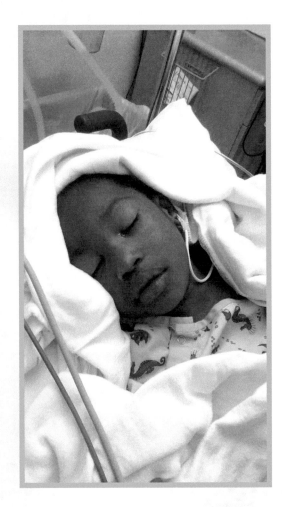

She's always in and out of the hospital so she became very close to a doctor by the name of Mr. Paw who's been there every step of the way and on the days she had to visit him she will get up very very early to get ready because she was very excited that she was able to see one of her great friends....

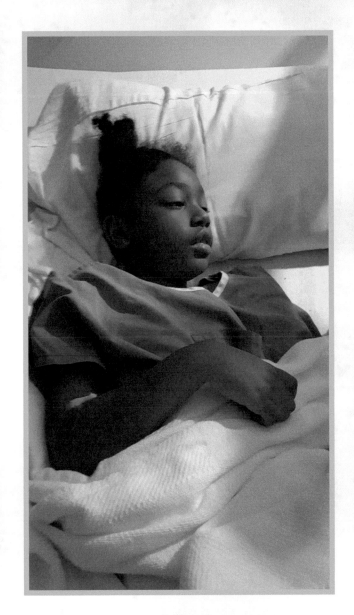
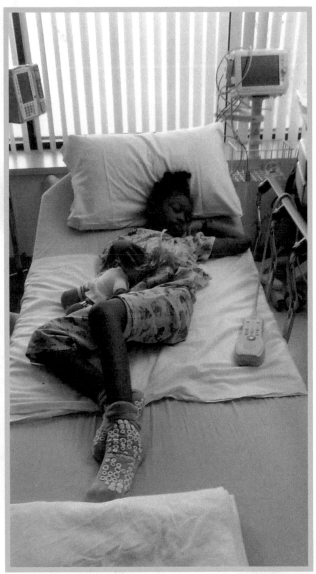

False will get out of bed, brush her teeth with the help of her grandmother whose name is Linda, who is also very close to. False love for her granny to do almost everything with her and she really love for her to get her together to see Dr. Paws on the days she had a doctor's appointment....

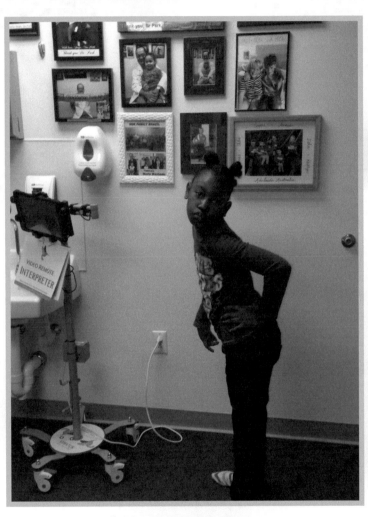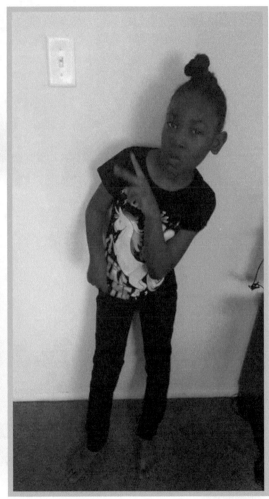

Dr. Paws: Hey False, how are you today?

False: Aw, well I am doing just fine and I brought you a gift Dr. Paws!

Dr. Paws: That is so sweet False! I keep all my gifts you give me on my desk right next to me!

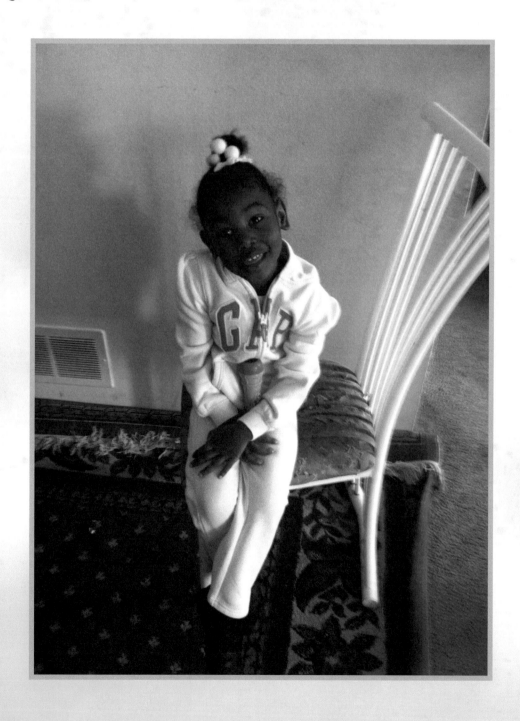

False was doing better and better from a surgery she had months ago due to her having epilepsy and cerebral palsy.

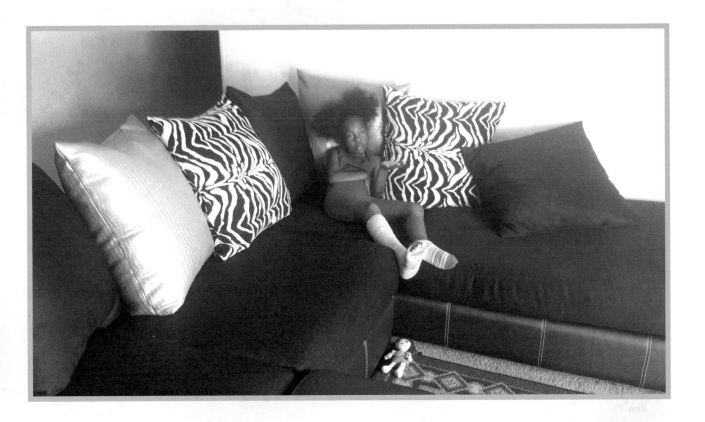

At the beginning, it was a challenge for her but still she will still smile and wiggle the parts of her body she was able to move.

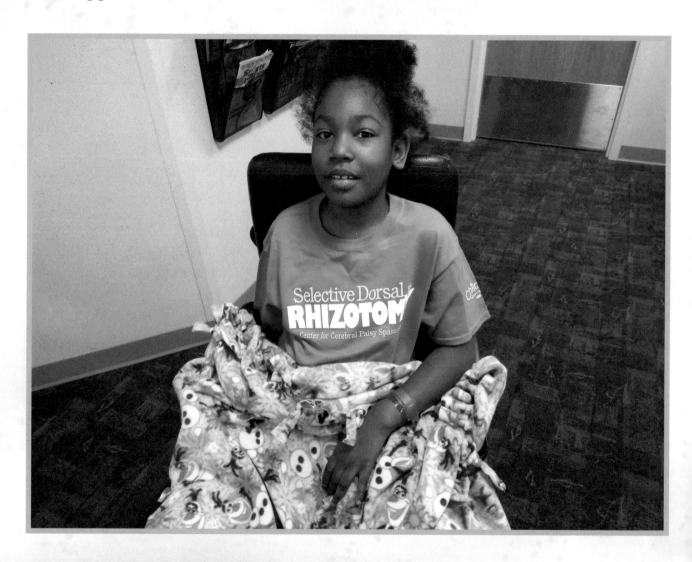

As she got better her mother Shine will take her to different places around the area to see her friends which everyone loved to see False and her mother visit....

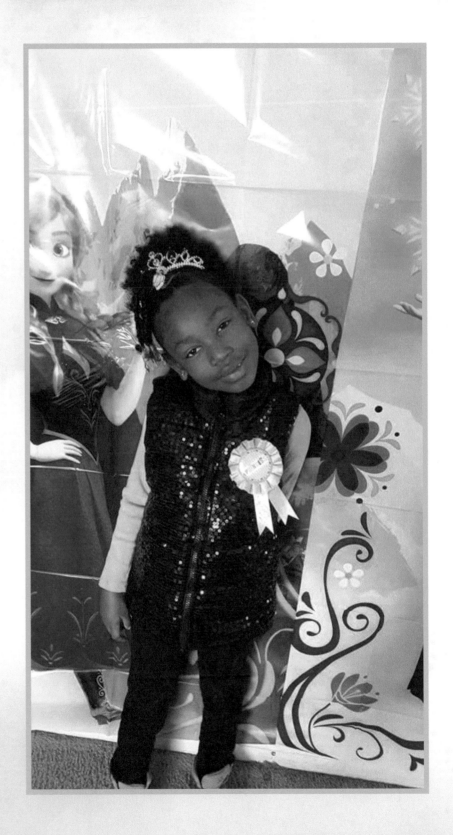

Her grandmother Linda will laugh and laugh because she loves to see False act her silly ways because it showed her. She was feeling just fine that day even though some days, False will sleep all day from her putting so much energy into the day before.

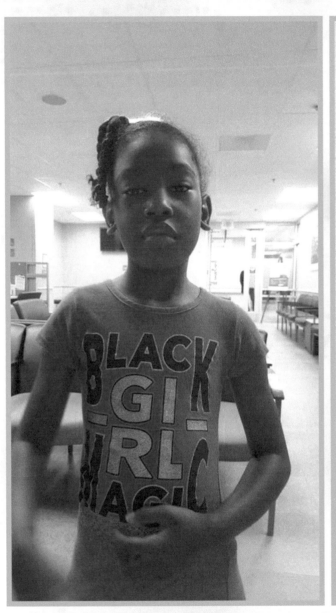 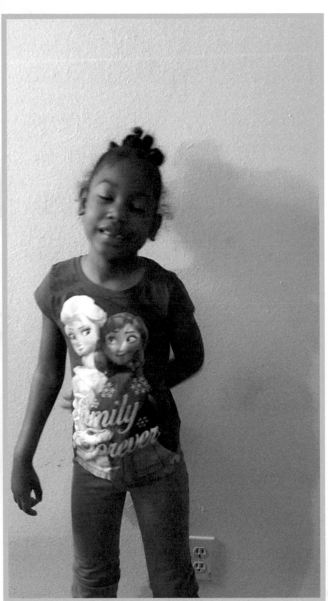

At the age of six, False had brain surgery that made her go to physical therapy twice a week. Oh how she will cry and cry because she disliked the way the doctor will make her do different things to get her strength back....BUT STILL THAT SMILE WILL BE THERE....

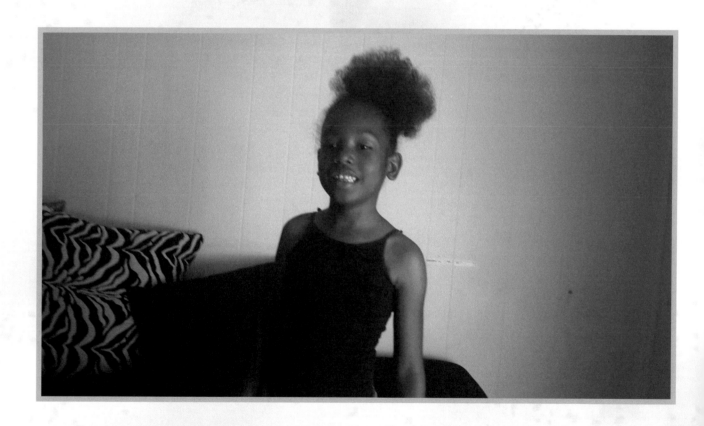

False was ONE out of the three people in the world that had a special surgery to help her develop a lil better with her mobility to move forward in life. But as we all know that false is also a very very strong princess. So she progressed very well....

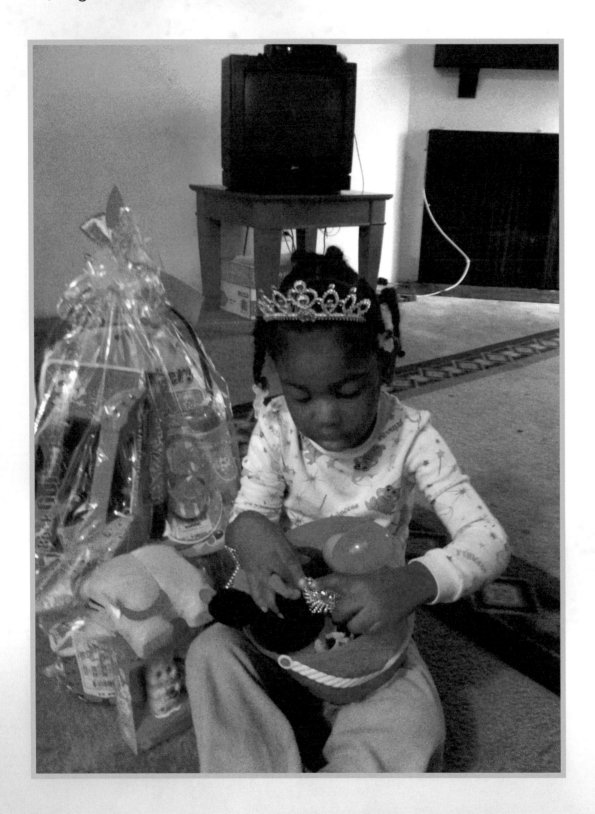

But as time go on, False was more and more in need which she was given a nurse who comes by every week and who comes by everyday.... She also will be given therapy twice a week where she will learn how to walk on her on without a help and do other things as far as bathing, eating and so much more......

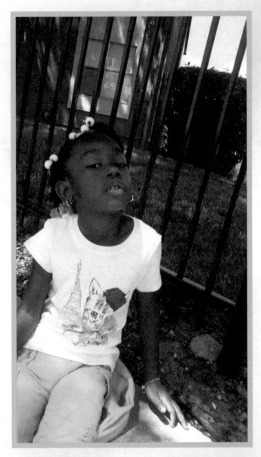
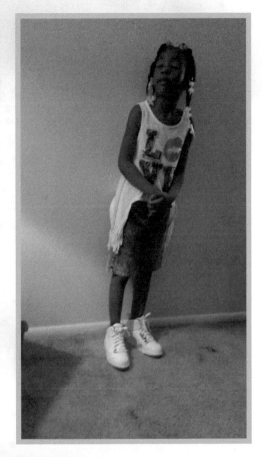
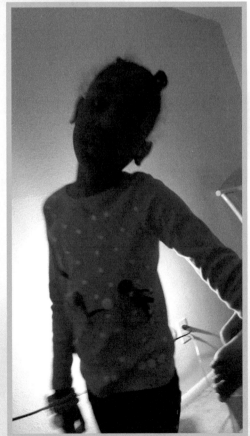

There are a lot of people in the world but only a few with the health that False has.....For some, it will seem that many people won't care about the special needs that False has. So there were a lot of questions....But even False will tell it all. She will tell you, from the beginning to this day, she still stands tall now!!

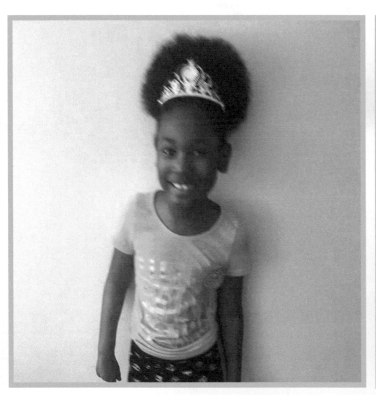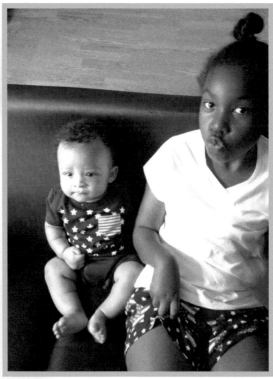

Printed in the United States
By Bookmasters